WATER AEROBICS WORKOUT FOR SENIORS

STRENGTHEN YOUR MUSCLES AND IMPROVE YOUR BALANCE

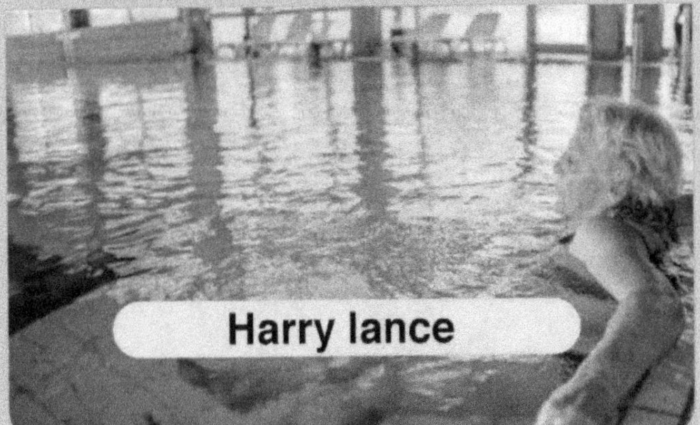

Abstract

The Water Aerobics Workout Plan offers a refreshing and effective fitness regimen designed for individuals seeking low-impact yet high-intensity exercises. This 100-word abstract encapsulates the plan's key features.

Dive into a 14-day aquatic adventure that harnesses water's buoyancy and resistance to sculpt a healthier you. With a focus on cardiovascular conditioning, strength building, and flexibility enhancement, this plan caters to all fitness levels. The water's gentle support minimizes joint strain, making it ideal for those with mobility issues or joint discomfort. Dive into dynamic movements, from water jogging to aqua lunges, and feel the burn without the impact.

Whether you're a beginner or a seasoned aquatic enthusiast, this plan provides a structured approach to improve fitness, boost endurance, and enhance overall well-being. Jump into the pool and embark on a journey to a healthier, more vibrant you.

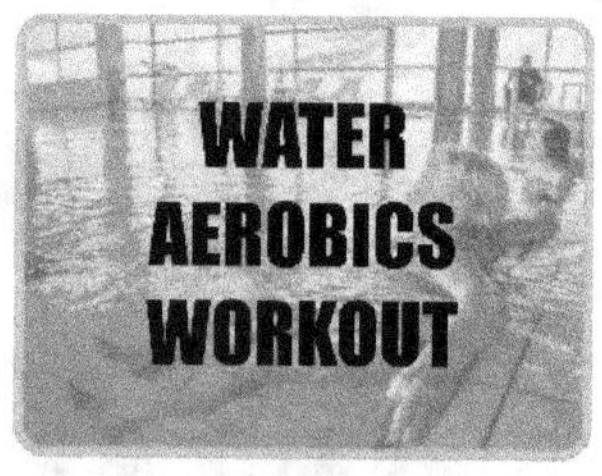

TABLE OF CONTENTS

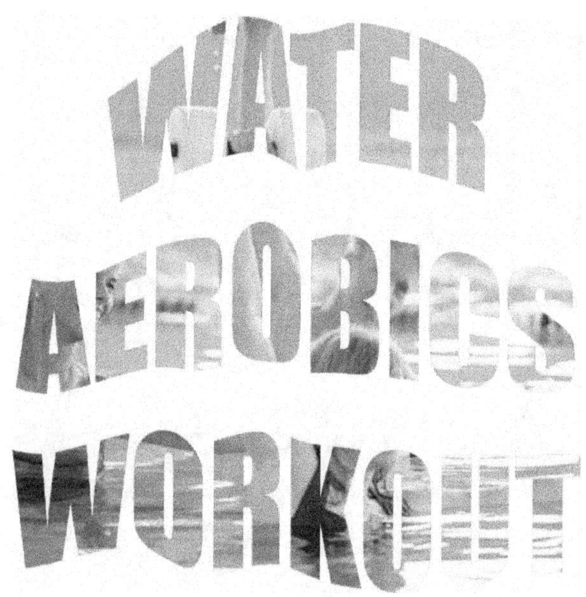
WATER
AEROBICS
WORKOUT

Mark's Story

Mark had always been skeptical about fitness plans, but when his doctor recommended water aerobics to ease his joint pain, he decided to give it a shot. He stumbled upon a 14-day water aerobics workout plan online and committed himself to it.

The first day was tough. He struggled to keep up with the movements and felt like a fish out of water. However, he refused to give up. Mark persevered, day after day. With each passing session, he grew stronger, more flexible, and confident in the water.

By the end of the 14 days, Mark was amazed at the transformation. His joint pain had subsided, and he felt more energetic than ever. Not only did he complete the workout plan, but he also exceeded it. He had discovered a newfound love for water aerobics and continued to incorporate it into his daily routine.

Mark's success story became an inspiration for others, proving that with determination and the right plan, anyone can achieve their fitness goals.

Day 1: Water Aerobics

1. Warm-up exercises

Certainly! Warm-up exercises for seniors are important to prepare the body for more strenuous activity and reduce the risk of injury. Here's a step-by-step guide for a gentle warm-up routine suitable for seniors:

1. Deep Breathing (2-3 minutes): Start by standing or sitting comfortably. Inhale deeply through your nose, expanding your chest, and exhale slowly through your mouth. Repeat several times to increase oxygen flow and relax.

2. Neck Rotations (1 minute): Gently rotate your neck in a clockwise and then counterclockwise direction. Be slow and deliberate, avoiding any sudden movements.

3. Shoulder Rolls (1 minute): Roll your shoulders forward and backward in a circular motion to loosen up the shoulder muscles.

4. Arm Circles (1 minute): Extend your arms out to the sides and move them in both directions in tiny, controlled circles. This gets your shoulder joints warmed up.

5. Wrist and Ankle Circles (1 minute each): Gently rotate your wrists and ankles to improve mobility and circulation in these joints.

6. Hip Marches (1 minute): While standing, lift your knees alternately towards your chest in a slow marching motion. Hold onto a sturdy surface for balance if needed.

7. Knee Lifts (1 minute): Stand upright and lift one knee towards your chest, then switch to the other. This helps warm up your hip and knee joints.

8. Leg Swings (1 minute each leg): Hold onto a stable surface for balance and swing one leg forward and backward, then switch to the other leg. This loosens up the hip joints.

9. Calf Raises (1 minute): Stand with your feet hip-width apart and slowly rise up onto your toes, then lower your heels back down. This strengthens your calf muscles.

10. Gentle Arm and Leg Stretches (2 minutes): Perform gentle stretches for your arms, legs, and back. Hold each stretch for about 15-30 seconds, but don't push yourself too hard.

11. Walking in Place (2-3 minutes): Finish your warm-up by walking in place at a comfortable pace. This gradually increases your heart rate and body temperature.

12. Cool Down: After your activity, don't forget to cool down with some static stretches to maintain flexibility and reduce muscle soreness.

Always pay attention to your body's signals and adjust these workouts as necessary. Before beginning a new workout regimen, it's a good idea to speak with a healthcare professional if you have any underlying health ailments or concerns.

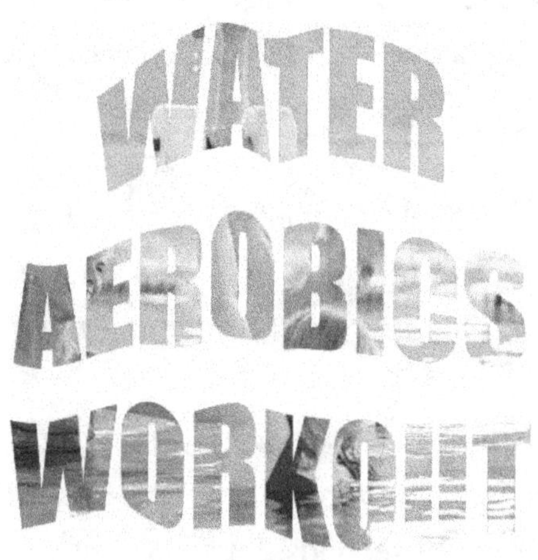

2.Gentle water walking

Gentle water walking can be a great exercise for seniors. Here are step-by-step instructions to get started:

Consult Your Doctor: Before starting any new exercise routine, it's important to check with your doctor, especially if you have any medical conditions or concerns.

1. Choose the Right Pool: Look for a pool that offers water at a comfortable temperature. A heated pool is often best for seniors.

2. Proper Attire: Wear appropriate swimwear and water shoes with good traction to prevent slipping.

3. Warm-Up: Begin with some gentle stretches on the pool deck to warm up your muscles.

4. Enter the Water Slowly: Walk slowly into the water to acclimate your body to the temperature. Start with water at waist level.

5. Maintain Good Posture: Stand up straight, engage your core muscles, and keep your shoulders relaxed.

6. Start Walking: Begin walking in the water. You can start with walking forward and then try walking backward. Focus on taking slow, deliberate steps.

7. Control Your Breathing: Pay attention to your breathing. Inhale through your nose and exhale through your mouth in a relaxed manner.

8. Use Buoyancy: Take advantage of the water's buoyancy to reduce the impact on your joints. You can also use flotation devices if needed.

9. Gradual Progress: Start with short sessions, around 10-15 minutes, and gradually increase the time as you become more comfortable and confident.

10. Cool Down: After your water walk, cool down with some more gentle stretches in the water.

11. Keep Hydrated: It's crucial to keep hydrated, even while you're in the water. Before and after your workout, drink some water.

12. Take Note of Your Body: Be mindful of how your body is feeling. If you feel pain or discomfort, halt and take a break.

13. Consistency: Aim for regular sessions, ideally 3-4 times
    a week, to experience the full benefits of water walking.

Enjoy the Experience: Water walking should be an enjoyable
and low-impact way to stay active. Have fun and socialize
with others if you're in a group setting.

Remember, the key is to start slowly and progress at your
own pace. If you're unsure about any aspect of water
walking, consider working with a qualified instructor who
can provide guidance and support tailored to your needs

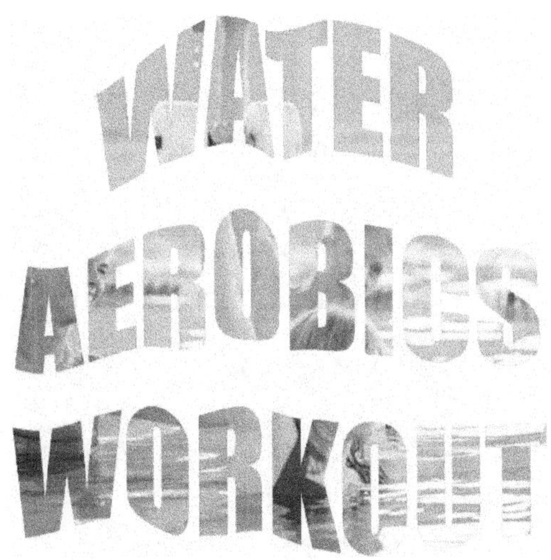

3. Arm circles and stretches

Starting arm circles and stretches for seniors is an excellent way to improve flexibility and mobility while promoting joint health. Begin by standing or sitting comfortably with good posture.

1.Arm Circles

- At shoulder height, extend your arms out to the sides.

- Gently rotate your arms in small circles, gradually increasing the size.

- Do this for 30 seconds in each direction (clockwise and counterclockwise). Maintain slow, controlled movements to avoid strain.

2.Shoulder Stretches

With your opposite hand, gently grasp the arm that is raised across your chest.

Hold for 15 to 30 seconds while allowing your shoulder to expand. Then switch sides once again.

3.Tricep Stretch:

- Raise one arm overhead and bend your elbow, reaching your hand down your back.

- Hold your bent elbow with your opposite hand and gently pull. Hold for 15-30 seconds, then switch sides.

4.Wrist and Forearm Stretches

- Put one arm out in front of you, palm up.

- Pull your fingers down gradually with your opposing hand.

- Switch after 15 to 30 seconds of holding.

- 5.Repeat 2-4 times:
- To increase flexibility, repeat each stretch 2-4 times on each side.

5.Cool down and relaxation

Cooling down after physical activity is crucial for the body's recovery. It involves gradually reducing exercise intensity to return the heart rate and breathing to normal.

This helps prevent dizziness and muscle cramps. But cooling down isn't just physical; it's also about mental relaxation.

Spend a few minutes doing some light stretching after working out. This releases tension and lengthens muscles. Also crucial is deep breathing. Deeply inhale through the nose, hold for a moment, and then slowly exhale through the mouth. This eases mental tension and lowers stress.

Cooling down isn't limited to exercise; it's a life practice. It's about finding moments of tranquility in our fast-paced world, promoting both physical and mental well-being.

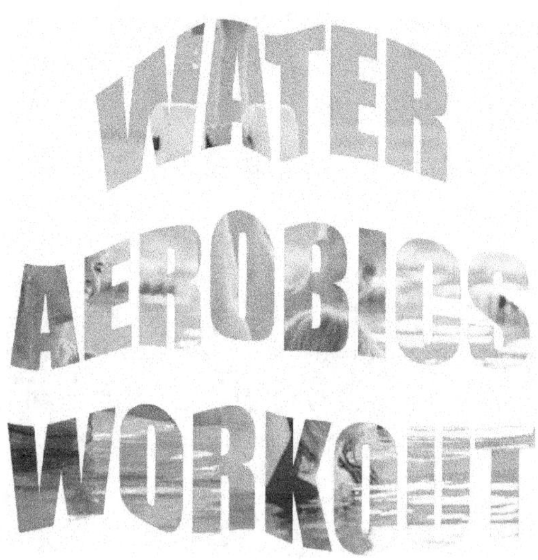

4.Leg lifts and kicks

Yes, I can help you with that. Leg lifts and kicks can be beneficial for seniors to improve leg strength and flexibility.

Here's a simple way to start:

1.Warm-up

Begin with a gentle warm-up to prepare your muscles. March in place or take a
short walk for about 5 minutes.

2.Chair Leg Lifts:

- Put your feet level on the ground and sit upright on a firm chair.
- For balance, cling to the chair's sides.
- Keep your toes pointing up and lift one leg straight out in front of you.
- Hold for a few while before bringing it back down. Repeat on each leg 10 to 15 times.

3.Standing Leg Kicks

- Use a tabletop or a chair as support as you stand there.

- Hold onto the chair or countertop for balance.
- Slowly lift one leg straight behind you, keeping your toes pointed forward.
- Kick your leg back gently and lower it.
- Repeat for 10-15 times on each leg.

Cool Down: Finish with a cool-down by walking in place or performing gentle stretches for your legs.

Remember to go at your own pace and only do what feels comfortable. If you have any existing medical conditions or concerns, it's a good idea to consult with a healthcare professional before starting a new exercise routine.

5. Wall-supported squats

Certainly! Wall-supported squats are a great exercise for seniors to improve leg strength and stability. Here's how to start:

1.Warm-up: Begin with a gentle warm-up to prepare your muscles. March in place or take a short walk for about 5 minutes.

2. Find a Wall

- Place your back against a strong wall as you stand.
- Maintain a foot-wide distance between your feet and the wall.

3.Proper Squat Form

- Place your hands on your hips or hold onto a stable surface like a chair for balance. Slowly lower your body by bending your knees and hips as if you're sitting back into an imaginary chair.

- Keep your back straight, chest up, and gaze forward.
- Lower yourself as far as you comfortably can, ideally until your thighs are parallel to the ground or as close as possible.

4. Hold and Rise

For a little period, stay in the squat position while keeping your balance against the wall.

To stand back up, drive through your heels and tighten your leg muscles. As you ascend, exhale.

5.Repetitions:

Start with sets of 5–10 repetitions.

Increase the amount of repetitions progressively as you get stronger and more at ease.

6.Cool Down: Finish with a cool-down by walking in place or performing gentle leg stretches.

6.Water jogging

Water jogging is an excellent low-impact exercise for seniors, as it provides buoyancy and reduces stress on the joints. Here's how to start:

1.Find a Suitable Pool

- Look for a pool with a depth that allows you to comfortably stand or perform water jogging. A heated pool can be more comfortable for seniors.

2.Warm-up:

- Begin with a few minutes of walking in the water to warm up your muscles.

3.Proper Water Depth

- Ensure the water is at chest or waist level, depending on your height and comfort.

4.Jogging Motion

- In the water, keep your head up.
- To begin, jog with your knees slightly up while taking little steps.
- Maintain a tight core and a straight back.
- Keep your arms in the water while jogging with them as if you were on land.

5.Start Slowly

- Start by running in the water for 5–10 minutes.
- As your endurance increases, gradually lengthen the exercise.

6.Water Resistance

- Remember that water provides resistance, which can help improve muscle strength over time.

7.Cool Down

- After your water jogging session, cool down with a few minutes of walking in the water at a slower pace.

8.Safety Precautions

- Always be aware of your surroundings in the pool.
- Use a flotation device or belt if needed for added support and safety.

9.Consult with a Professional

If you're new to water exercise or have any medical concerns, it's a good idea to consult with a
healthcare professional or a certified aquatic fitness instructor for guidance and to ensure that water jogging is safe for you.

Water jogging is a gentle and effective way to improve cardiovascular fitness, leg strength, and overall well-being for seniors while minimizing impact on the joints.

Cool down and relaxation

Cooling down after exercise is crucial for recovery. It involves gentle, low-intensity movements and stretches that help reduce heart rate and ease muscles. Cooling down can enhance flexibility, prevent muscle soreness, and promote relaxation. Focus on deep breathing and stretching major muscle groups, holding each stretch for 15-30 seconds. This routine aids in dissipating exercise-induced tension, leaving you feeling refreshed and rejuvenated.

7.Water resistance exercises

1. Certainly! Water resistance exercises are a great option for seniors because they are gentle on the joints while providing an effective workout. Here's how to get started:

2. Pick the Right Place: Look for a local pool or aquatic center that provides senior citizens open swim periods or water workout sessions. The ideal water temperature is between 84 and 88 degrees Fahrenheit (29 and 31 degrees Celsius).

3. Adopt the Proper Swimwear: Choose swimwear that is both comfy and flexible. Having traction on the pool floor can be helped by wearing water shoes with non-slip soles.

4. Warm Up First: Start your workout with a little warm-up in the water. You may relax your muscles by taking a walk in the water or performing gentle leg swings.

5. Use Buoyancy Aids: If necessary, you can use buoyancy aids during workouts to help with balance and support, such as foam noodles or water weights.

6. Pay attention to range of motion: Since water naturally offers resistance, even easy exercises like leg lifts and arm circles can be beneficial. Increase the range of motion and flexibility of your joints.

7. Pay close attention to your breathing. Use your nose to take in air, and your mouth to let it out. This is critical to ensuring optimum oxygen flow when exercising.

8. Balance and Posture: Work on your balance by walking heel to toe or standing on one leg in the water. In order to prevent tension, good posture is crucial.

9. Building Strength: Work on your strength by using the water's resistance. Try workouts like arm curls, leg lifts, water squats, and water walking. Start with a small number of repetitions and increase them as you get more comfortable.

10. Cool Down: To reduce muscular discomfort, stretch out gently in the water after your workout.

11. Even if you're in the water, it's still important to keep hydrated. Drink more water as necessary.

12. Pay Attention to Your Body: During and after each session, pay close attention to how your body feels. Stop and see your doctor if you feel any pain or discomfort.

13. Consistency is Key: Aim for frequent sessions to get the most out of water resistance workouts. A excellent place to start is once or twice each week.

8. Floating noodle workouts

Certainly! Floating noodle workouts are a fun and effective way to exercise in the water while providing buoyancy and resistance. Here's how to start:

Get the Right Equipment
A pool noodle or a few pool noodles are required. Usually, they are large foam cylinders that float in the water.

For more traction and comfort, water shoes can also be a good idea. Choose the Proper Location:

Find a pool with water that is deep enough for your feet to touch the bottom while you can float comfortably in it. Warm-Up:

Warming up gradually should precede your workout. For a few minutes, walk or tread water to warm up your muscles.

9. Floating Position

Floating noodle workouts are a fun and effective way to exercise in the water while providing buoyancy and resistance. Here's how to start:

1.Get the Right Equipment

- You'll need a pool noodle or a few pool noodles. These are typically long foam cylinders that provide buoyancy in the water.
- You might also want water shoes for added traction and comfort.

2.Select the Right Location

- Find a pool with water deep enough to allow you to float comfortably while your feet can touch the pool floor.

3.Warm-Up

- Start your workout with a gentle warm-up. Walk or tread water for a few minutes to get your muscles ready.

4. Floating Position

- To begin, hold the pool noodle under your arms and allow your body to float horizontally in the water.
- Keep your head above water to breathe comfortably.

5.Core Exercises

- Engage your core muscles to maintain balance and stability as you perform various exercises.
- Try exercises like leg lifts, bicycle kicks, or scissor kicks to work on your abdominal muscles.

6. Arm Exercises

- Extend your arms along the length of the pool noodle and perform arm movements such as bicep curls, tricep extensions, or lateral raises for shoulder strength.

7. Leg Exercises

Hold the noodle with your hands for balance and do leg exercises like flutter kicks or frog kicks to target your leg muscles.

8.Cardiovascular Exercises

- Incorporate movements that get your heart rate up. For example, you can do jumping jacks or cross-country skiing movements with the noodle.

9. Balance and Coordination

- Challenge your balance by standing on one leg on the noodle or trying to sit on it while maintaining stability.

10. Cool Down

- After your workout, spend a few minutes floating on the noodle to relax your muscles and cool down.

11. Safety First

- Always be cautious in the water, especially if you're trying new exercises. Make sure you're in a pool with a lifeguard or someone who can assist if needed.

12. Stay Hydrated

- Keep yourself hydrated even while you're in the water. Drink more water as necessary.

13.Gradual Progression:

- Start with simple exercises and gradually increase the intensity and complexity of your routine as you become more comfortable and confident in the water

10. Water bicycle

Water biking, also known as aqua cycling, is a low-impact exercise that can be suitable for seniors. Here's how to get started with water biking for seniors:

1. Choose the Right Pool:

- Look for a pool or aquatic facility that offers water biking classes or has water bikes available for use. Ensure the water is at a comfortable temperature, usually around 84-88 degrees Fahrenheit (29-31 degrees Celsius).

2. Proper Attire

- Wear appropriate swimwear, and consider aqua shoes for better traction on the bike's pedals.

3. Adjust the Bike

- If you're using a water bike, ask for assistance to adjust the bike's seat and handlebars to a comfortable height. Proper bike adjustment is crucial for comfort and safety.

4.Mounting the Bike

- Approach the water bike from the pool deck or a poolside platform. Hold onto the bike's handles and carefully straddle the seat before sitting down.

5.Starting Pedaling

- Begin pedaling slowly to get used to the motion. Water provides natural resistance, so adjust your pedaling speed and resistance level based on your comfort and fitness level.

6. Posture

- Keep a straight spine when bicycling. Avoid slouching, keep your back upright, and activate your core.

7.Vary the Intensity

- As you become more comfortable, you can increase the intensity of your workout by pedaling faster or adding resistance if your water bike allows for it.

8. Balancing

- Balancing on a water bike can be different from a regular bicycle, so take your time to get accustomed to it. Hold onto the handles for stability if needed.

9. Safety

- Always exercise caution. If you feel unsteady or experience any discomfort, stop pedaling and stabilize yourself before continuing.

10. Duration:

- Start with shorter sessions, perhaps 15-20 minutes, and gradually increase the duration as your fitness improves.

11. Cool Down:

- After your water biking session, take a few minutes to cool down by pedaling slowly and stretching your legs in the water.

12. Stay Hydrated

- Even though you're in the water, it's important to stay hydrated. Take water breaks as needed.

13. Consistency

- Aim for regular water biking sessions to experience the full benefits. A few times a week can be a good starting point.

14. Enjoy the Experience

- Water biking can be a refreshing and enjoyable way to exercise. Focus on having fun while staying active.

Remember that water biking is a gentle and joint-friendly exercise, making it suitable for seniors. However, it's essential to listen to your body, start slowly, and progress at your own pace. If you're new to water biking, consider taking a class or seeking guidance from a qualified instructor to ensure a safe and effective workout.

Cool down and relaxation

After a vigorous workout or physical activity, it's tempting to head straight for the showers or rush off to your next task. However, taking the time to cool down and relax is an essential part of any fitness routine. Not only does it provide physical benefits, but it also promotes mental and emotional well-being.

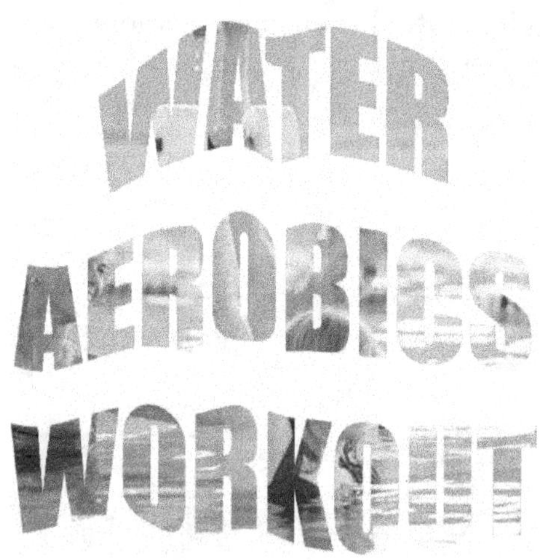

11. Water jogging intervals

Water jogging can be a great low-impact exercise for seniors. To start water jogging intervals, follow these steps:

1. Find a Pool

- Look for a pool with water that's chest to shoulder deep, ideally heated for comfort.

2.Warm-Up

- Start with a gentle warm-up by walking in the water for about 5-10 minutes to loosen up your muscles.

3. Interval Basics

- Water jogging intervals involve alternating between periods of higher and lower intensity. This can be done by adjusting your jogging speed.

4.High-Intensity Phase

- Jog in place or move around the pool at a faster pace for 1-2 minutes. You should feel your heart rate increase during this phase.

5. Low-Intensity Phase

- Slow down to a comfortable pace or even walk in the water for 1-2 minutes to recover.

6. Repeat:

- Alternate between high and low-intensity phases for a total of 20-30 minutes. Start with shorter intervals and gradually increase the duration as your fitness improves.

7. Cool Down

- Finish your workout with 5-10 minutes of gentle walking in the water to gradually lower your heart rate.

8. Stretch

- Perform some gentle stretching exercises to improve flexibility and reduce muscle tension.

9. Hydrate

- Remember to stay hydrated by drinking water before, during, and after your water jogging session.

10. Take Note of Your Body

- Be mindful of how your body is feeling. Stop doing anything right away and seek medical advice if you feel any pain or discomfort.

- Aim to water jog 2-3 times a week to build endurance and strength over time.

Remember, safety is the top priority. Adjust the intensity and duration of your intervals based on your fitness level and how you feel during the workout. It's also a good idea to have a lifeguard or someone nearby when doing water exercises, especially if you're a senior.

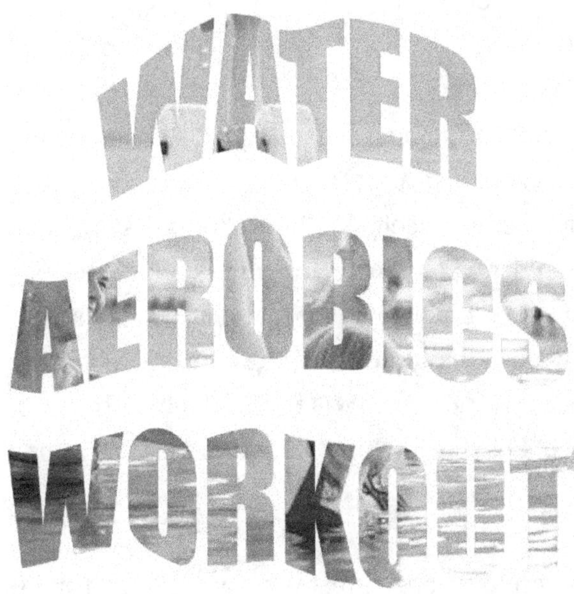

12: Core Strengthening

1. Standing Twists:

Twists performed while standing are a great technique to warm up your core and increase spinal mobility. Put your feet hip-width apart to start out. Continue to hold your arms out in front of you, parallel to the floor. Engage your core muscles as you slowly turn your torso to one side. After a little period of holding the twist, come back to the center. On the opposite side, repeat. This workout helps you get better balance and gets your body ready for harder exercises. b.

2. Water Planks:

A version of the standard plank exercise that you may do in the water is called a water plank. Submerge yourself and float on your stomach. With your elbows exactly behind your shoulders, place your forearms on the water's surface. To keep your body in a straight line from head to heels, engage your core, glutes, and legs. For as long as you can, maintain this posture. Water resistance offers a special challenge, boosting stability and tightening up your core. c.

3. Poolside Stretches

Poolside stretches are a great way to cool down and improve flexibility after a workout. Stand by the pool's edge and hold onto it for support. Perform stretches like leg swings, quad stretches, or calf stretches. The buoyancy of the water reduces the risk of overstretching and provides a soothing environment for post-workout relaxation.

4. Cool Down and Relaxation:

Take five to ten minutes to calm down and unwind after your workout . After taking a gentle walk to lower your heart rate, practice deep breathing. Gently stretch while sitting or lying down by reaching for your toes or turning your ankles. This stage facilitates muscle healing, lowers the possibility of discomfort, and fosters a feeling of calm and wellbeing.

Remember to adapt these exercises to your fitness level and consult with a fitness professional if you're new to aquatic workouts. While the explanations above are concise, always prioritize safety and proper form during your exercise routine

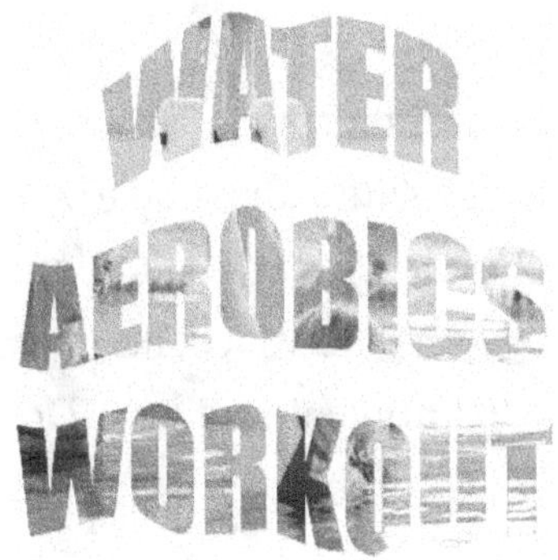

13: Flexibility and Range of Motion

Flexibility and range of motion are vital for seniors' well-being. Regular stretching exercises can enhance joint mobility, reduce stiffness, and prevent falls. These activities, like yoga or gentle stretches, improve balance and posture, ensuring seniors maintain independence and enjoy an active, pain-free lifestyle in their golden years.

1 .Gentle Stretches:

 Start your senior workout with gentle stretches to warm up your muscles. These can include neck rolls, shoulder stretches, and ankle circles. Hold each stretch for about 15-30 seconds, breathing deeply. This helps improve flexibility, reduces the risk of injury, and prepares your body for more intense movements.

2. Arm and Leg Circles

Arm and leg circles are fantastic for seniors. For arms, extend them out to the sides and make slow, controlled circles in both directions. For legs, stand and lift one leg, making gentle circles with your foot. This exercise enhances joint mobility and helps prevent stiffness. Do 10-15 circles in each direction for each limb.

Tai Chi is a low-impact workout. The buoyancy of the water provides resistance while reducing joint stress. This mild martial art uses fluid movements to increase flexibility, strength, and balance. To learn fundamental Tai Chi techniques in the water, watch a video or listen to an instructor. Seniors who have joint problems would notably benefit from it.

4 .Take five to ten minutes to calm down and unwind after your workout After taking a gentle walk to lower your heart rate, practice deep breathing. Gently stretch while sitting or lying down by reaching for your toes or turning your ankles. This stage facilitates muscle healing, lowers the possibility of discomfort, and fosters a feeling of calm and wellbeing.

Incorporating these components into a senior workout routine can help maintain and improve flexibility, range of motion, and overall physical health while keeping exercises safe and enjoyable. Always consult a healthcare professional before starting a new exercise program, especially if you have pre-existing health conditions.

14: Rest and Recovery

1. Breathing Exercises for Seniors

Seniors must do breathing exercises to improve their lungs' capacity, oxygenate their bodies, and lessen stress. Breathing through the diaphragm is one common method. Seniors should find a comfortable position to sit or lay down in, with one hand on the abdomen and the other on the chest.

Deeply inhale through the nose, letting the belly rise, and then slowly exhale through pursed lips. This regular activity enhances lung function and encourages calm.

2. Gentle Floating for Seniors

A low-impact water aerobics activity that is perfect for elders is gentle floating. In a pool or shallow water, it calls for gradual movements. Senior individuals can kick lightly, do arm circles, and elevate their legs.

Joint sprains and injuries are less likely because of the resistance and buoyancy that water offers. It's an excellent technique to increase joint comfort while enhancing cardiovascular health, flexibility, and muscular strength.

Seniors who use mindful relaxation techniques can reduce stress and enhance their mental health. Progressive muscular relaxation is one useful method. Seniors who are seated or lying down concentrate on each muscle area, tension it for a little period of time, and then release it while concentrating on the relaxation sensation. This encourages mental and physical relaxation, lessens anxiety, and improves the quality of sleep.

Seniors need to perform restorative stretches frequently to keep their flexibility and mobility. The sitting hamstring stretch is a common stretches. Seniors lean forward from the hips, maintaining their backs straight, while they sit on the edge of a chair and stretch one leg forward. After holding for 15 to 30 seconds, switch to the other leg. This exercise preserves range of motion while preventing muscular stiffness.

Seniors should always get advice from a doctor or trainer before beginning any new exercise program, particularly if they have underlying medical issues. These exercises may be modified for individual requirements and fitness levels to provide seniors with a safe and efficient training program..

15: Low-Impact Aerobics

1. Water Aerobics Routines

Water aerobics is like dancing in the pool! You stand in the water, and we move our arms and legs to the music. It's like a fun workout party, and it's easy on your joints because the water supports you. We do exercises like leg kicks and arm circles. It's great for staying healthy and having fun with friends!

2.Water Marching

Water marching is just like marching in a parade, but in the pool. We stand up straight, lift our knees high, and move them up and down like we're marching. The water makes it a bit harder, but it's also gentle on our bodies. It's a fun way to build strong legs and stay fit while splashing around in the water.

3.Side Leg Lifts

Imagine you're a superhero, and you want to lift your leg to the side like you're flying. In the water, we do this exercise by standing tall and lifting one leg out to the side, then the other leg. It's like making big splashes with your feet. This helps make our legs strong and flexible.

After all the fun exercises, it's time to relax. We stand in the water, take deep breaths, and let our bodies float a bit. It's like being in a giant bathtub. We can stretch our arms and legs gently and feel how nice and calm the water makes us. This part is super important to keep our bodies happy and relaxed.

So, in water aerobics, we dance, march, lift our legs, and then have a nice, relaxing time in the water. It's like a fun adventure in the pool that keeps us healthy and happy

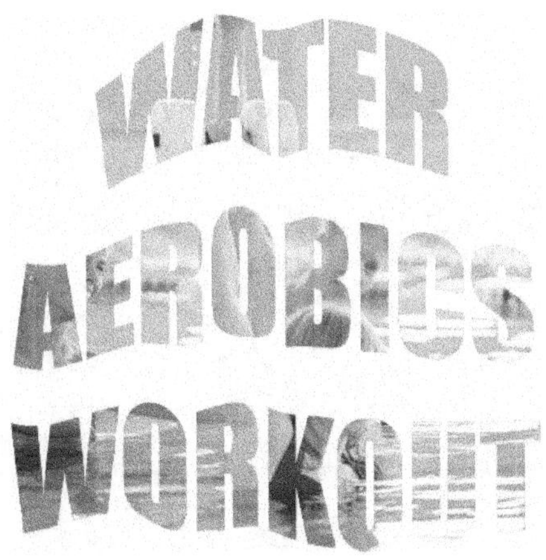

16: Strength and Endurance

1. Resistance Band Exercises

Resistance band exercises are like magic rubber ropes that help keep your muscles strong. They are colorful and stretchy. Seniors can sit or stand while using them.

- **Bicep Curls:** Palms facing up, grasp the band with both hands. Bend your elbows as though you were bringing soup cans to your shoulders.

- **Leg Lifts:** With one foot, step on the band while holding the other end. As though you were marching, lift your leg to the side.

- **Seated Row:** Sit down, encircle your feet with the band, and draw the ends of the band toward your waist as if you were rowing a boat.

- **Overhead Press:** Stand on the band and lift it over your head, like lifting a big balloon.

2. Water Jogging with Intervals

Water jogging is like dancing in a swimming pool. It's gentle on your joints.

- **Warm-Up:** Walk slowly in the water to warm up, like you're taking a stroll.

- **Jogging:** Start jogging in the water, lifting your knees high. It's like jogging on the moon, but in water.

- **Interval Play:** Speed up and slow down your jogging like you're playing a game of stop and go.

3. Floating Dumbbell Exercises

Imagine doing exercises while floating on a cloud! Floating dumbbell exercises are done in the water, making them fun and gentle.

- **Water Weights** : Hold lightweight dumbbells in the water, and do arm lifts like you're hugging a big, fluffy teddy bear.

- **Leg Floats** : Lie on your back, let your legs float, and gently kick them like you're swimming in the sky.

- **12.Water Walk:** Walk in the water while holding dumbbells. It's like taking a walk on a cloud.

4. Cool Down and Relaxation

- After all that fun exercise, it's important to relax and cool down.

- Deep Breaths: Sit or lie down and take deep breaths, like you're blowing up a balloon.

- Stretch: Reach your arms up and stretch like you're waking up from a nap.

- Massage: Gently rub your muscles with your hands, like giving yourself a mini massage.

- Smile: Lastly, smile and be happy. You did a great job staying healthy!

- These aerobics workouts for seniors are like a playful adventure that keeps you strong, happy, and feeling great.
- So, grab your resistance band, head to the pool, or float on a cloud in the water – and don't forget to smile!

17: Cardio Mix

1. Water Aerobics Variations

Water aerobics is like dancing in the water. You move your arms and legs while standing in the pool. It's a fun way to exercise without putting too much pressure on your joints. You can do exercises like marching, kicking, and stretching. It's like a water dance party!

2. High Knees and Butt Kicks

High knees are like marching, but you lift your knees up high. It's like you're trying to touch your chest with your knees. Butt kicks are like jogging, but you try to kick your bottom with your heels. Both exercises make your legs strong and your heart happy.

3. Pool Volleyball

Pool volleyball is a game where you hit a ball over a net in the water. It's like regular volleyball, but you play in the pool, so you don't have to run as much. You can splash and have fun while trying to get the ball over the net. It's like a watery game of catch!

4. Cool Down and Relaxation

After all the fun exercises, it's important to cool down. You can stand in the water and move your arms gently like you're drawing big circles. Then, you can float on your back and relax, like you're taking a nap in the water. It helps your body and mind relax after all the excitement.

Remember, it's essential to be safe in the water and have someone there to watch you, like a lifeguard or a responsible grown-up. Water exercises are a great way for seniors to stay healthy and have a splashing good time

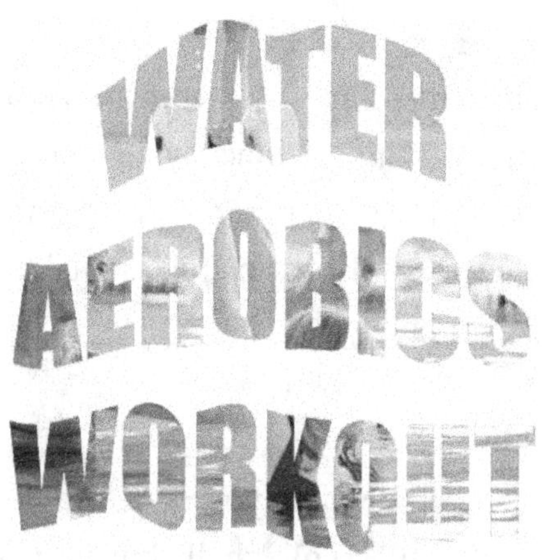

18: Balance and Coordination

1. Balance Exercises on One Leg

Imagine you're standing on one leg like a graceful flamingo. This is what balance exercises on one leg are like. They help seniors stay steady on their feet. Why is this important? Well, as we get older, sometimes our balance isn't as good as it used to be. These exercises make it stronger.

How to Do It:

- Stand Tall: Find a comfy spot. Lift one leg and stand on the other. Hold onto a chair or wall if needed.
- Tree Pose: Pretend to be a tree! Raise one foot onto the opposite leg's thigh and balance. Hold your hands in prayer pose.
- Airplane Pose: Like a superhero! Stretch one leg back and lean forward, keeping your arms out like wings.
- Count to 10: Try to balance for as long as you can. Count to 10, and then switch legs.

2. Water Yoga Poses:

Water yoga is like doing yoga in a giant pool. It's super gentle on your body, and the water helps you float and relax.

- Find a Pool: First, find a pool that's not too deep.
- Warm Up: Move your arms and legs gently in the water to warm up.
- Mountain Pose: Stand tall in the water, like a mountain. Reach your arms up to the sky and take deep breaths.
- Water Walk: Walk in the water, lifting your knees high. It's like walking on the moon!
- Floating Relax: Lay back and let the water hold you up. Close your eyes, and just float like a starfish.

3. Water Volleyball

Water volleyball is like regular volleyball, but you play it in the water. It's a fun way to exercise and cool off at the same time.

How to Do It:

- Get a Net: Set up a volleyball net in the pool or at the beach.
- Teams: Split into teams, and each team tries to get the ball over the net.
- Bump, Set, Spike: Use your hands to bump the ball, set it up, and then spike it over the net. Have Fun: The goal is to keep the ball from hitting the water on your side.

After all that exercising, it's important to cool down and relax, just like how you rest after playing a fun game.

How to Do It

- Locate a Quiet Place: Find a comfortable place to sit or to lie down.

- Deep Breathing: Inhale and exhale slowly and deeply. It's comparable like inflating a balloon and then deflating it.

- Stretching: To assist your muscles relax, gently stretch your arms, legs, and neck.

- Close your eyes and visualize a tranquil setting, such as a deserted beach or a lovely woodland. So there you have it!

Seniors may maintain their physical activity levels, have fun, and take care of themselves with activities like balance exercises, water yoga, water volleyball, and relaxation. Just keep in mind to relax and soak it all in.

19: Endurance Challenge

1.Longer Water Jogging Sessions:

Running on land, but in the water, is called water jogging. It's a mild form of exercise that has no negative effects on joints for elders.

More time in the water is spent during longer sessions, which is great for your heart and muscles. Think about walking in a pool while simultaneously moving your arms and legs to maintain balance.

This keeps you healthy and strengthens your heart. Therefore, when you hear the phrase "longer water jogging sessions," it simply refers to spending more time having fun in the water to keep in shape!

2. Deep Water Running

Running in deep water is like flopping around in the deep end of the pool while trying to run. To keep upright, you put on a special floaty belt. Because there is no stress on your knees or hips, it is incredibly mild on your body. It's like doing a magic trick without touching the earth! It may make you feel calm and content and is beneficial for your muscles.

3. Swim Laps or Water Dancing:

Comparable to swimming from one side of the pool to the other, lap swimming. It resembles a competitive race with oneself. To navigate the water, you use your arms and legs to paddle. Contrarily, water dance is similar to underwater dancing. While standing in the pool, you may wriggle, shake, and have a fantastic time dancing to the music. Both of them are enjoyable exercises that will strengthen your heart and body. It resembles a water party!

4. Cool Down and Relaxation

It's necessary to cool down and unwind after working out. Think of it like lowering the music player's volume after a dance party. You stretch or make gentle motions to assist your body relax. It's similar to praising your heart and muscles, "Great work! Let's now unwind. Following exercise, you should cool down and unwind to feel good and avoid pain.

Just like playing with your pals, these workouts are like water games and are a great way to keep in shape. Take pleasure in being in the water; it will keep you healthy and content.

20: Total Body Workout

- Seniors can benefit greatly from the low-impact exercise of water aerobics. It mixes strength and cardiovascular training in a mild, joint-friendly setting. Here is a straightforward procedure that can comprehend:

- Seniors can begin their warm-up exercises in the water by doing modest arm circles and leg swings. Think about swinging your arms in broad circles and swinging your legs like a pendulum. Joints and muscles are loosened up as a result.

- The next exercise is jogging. As you march, raise and lower your knees while standing in the water. This is heart-pumping exercise similar to a fun water jog.

- Leg lifts are now required. Lift one leg straight out in front of you while holding onto the side of the pool if necessary. After then, change to the opposite leg. It is comparable to raising your legs when swimming.

- Exercise your arms by simulating boat rowing. Put your feet in the water and sit on the side of the pool. Then, 'row' your arms like you would a boat. This strengthens your upper body and arms.

- Try standing on one leg to practice your balance. Lift one foot off the water's surface while holding onto the side of the pool if required. It's similar to a game of balancing.

- Stretch out gently to finish. Then, stoop to touch your toes by raising your arms high. Extend your arms and legs in every way.

2. Water Cycling for Seniors

- Seniors can increase their cardiovascular fitness and leg strength by participating in water cycling. Just picture pedaling a bike on the water! This is how it goes:

- Start in the pool's shallow end. Use a water bike or a floating mat if one is available. Move through the water by pedaling your legs as if you were riding a bicycle. It resembles cycling while fighting water resistance.

- Quicken your pedaling to make it more difficult. It feels like you're riding a real bike quicker!

- Keep your back straight, and tighten your abdominal muscles for stability. You want proper posture, much as when you ride a bike on the road.

3. Water Noodle Circuits for Seniors

- A pleasant aquatic obstacle course for seniors is what water noodle circuits are like. This is how it goes:

- To'swim' through the pool, kick your legs while holding on to a water noodle like it's a bar. It's like a race with water noodles!

- Now, twirl your body inside the noodle as if it were a hula hoop. It resembles a water hula hoop routine.

- The noodle may also be used as a jump rope. As it floats in the water, step over it. Jump roping in a swimming pool is how this works.

- Standing on one foot while holding the noodle in front of you will test your balance. It resembles a floating variation on a game of balance!

- After all that enjoyable activity, it's important to unwind and calm off. Imagine that it is now time to relax and sleep:

- A location in the pool with chest-deep water should be found. While remaining motionless, exhale deeply as though you were blowing out a candle and enjoying the scent of a lovely flower.

- Reaching for the stars, gently extend your arms and legs in the water. Your muscles will relax as a result.

- Paddle or leisurely stroll around the pool to stay cool. It's similar to going for a leisurely walk.

- To finish, float on your back and rely on the water to support you. Close your eyes, unwind, and savor the tranquility.

- These water exercises and relaxation techniques are not only great for seniors but also easy to understand, making them suitable for everyone.

Celebration and Reflection

1. Gentle Water Dance

Imagine older citizens performing gentle water dance in a pool, not just any dance! It resembles dancing as water sprays are all around you. Like when you play with water in a bathtub, the water is gentle on their body. Like when you walk gently while carrying a glass of water, it's neither too quick nor too difficult. It's an enjoyable method for elders to remain cool while exercising!

2. Cool Down and Relaxation

It's time to chill down and unwind after all the exercises. Imagine halting a rapid automobile and allowing it to cool. Seniors stretch gently and breathe deeply, just like you would when you were trying to relax. It's similar like pausing a movie, but with their body. It makes people feel content and at ease.

2. Setting Future Goals

Think of seniors as explorers going on a great journey. Setting objectives for the future is comparable to them determining where to go on their next excursion. They consider the goals they have for their workouts. It's similar to creating a birthday wish list. Seniors may like to increase their strength or learn new activities. It's like having exciting future plans!

To ensure that elders enjoy their workouts and maintain their health, keep in mind that making these explanations clear and enjoyable is the key.

Before beginning any new workout regimen, keep in mind to speak with a medical practitioner, especially if you have underlying medical issues. You may modify these workouts' time and intensity to meet your particular demands and degree of fitness. Enjoy the 14 days of water aerobics!

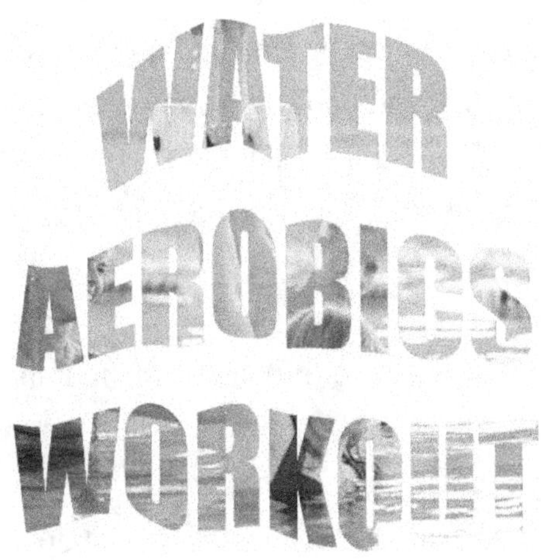

Conclusion

In conclusion, this Water Aerobics Workout Plan for Seniors offers a holistic approach to improving physical fitness, overall health, and well-being among older individuals. Through a carefully designed program that leverages the buoyancy and resistance of water, seniors can experience a wide array of benefits.

First and foremost, water aerobics is gentle on the joints, making it an ideal exercise choice for those dealing with arthritis or other musculoskeletal issues. It enhances cardiovascular endurance, promotes muscle strength and flexibility, and contributes to better balance and coordination all vital elements in maintaining independence as we age. Furthermore, the natural cooling effect of water reduces the risk of overheating, which can be a concern for seniors during regular workouts.

But it's not just about physical health; water aerobics can have a profoundly positive impact on mental and emotional well-being too. The social aspect of group classes fosters a sense of community and belonging, while the soothing properties of water can reduce stress and anxiety.

So, here's the motivation for you, dear reader: Embrace this Water Aerobics Workout Plan for Seniors as a path to rejuvenation and vitality. Let the gentle waters become your partners in fitness, guiding you towards a healthier and happier life. Remember, it's never too late to start, and with consistency and determination, you can experience the transformative power of water aerobics. So, jump in, make a splash, and embrace the joy of staying active and vibrant well into your golden years. Your body and mind will thank you for it, and you'll discover a newfound zest for life that you never thought possible. Dive in and make a splash, for your health and happiness await beneath the surface.

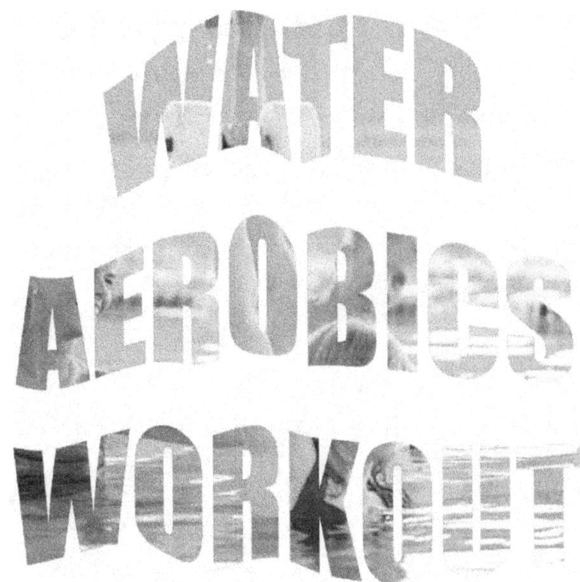

Thank you for taking the time to explore our Water Aerobics Workout Plan for Seniors. We're truly grateful for your interest in improving your health and well-being through water-based exercise. Your commitment to staying active and vibrant is inspiring.

Remember, age is just a number, and you have the power to make every splash count on your journey to a healthier and happier you. We hope this plan serves as a valuable resource in your quest for fitness and vitality.

If you have any questions or need further guidance, don't hesitate to reach out. We're here to support you every stroke of the way. Stay motivated, stay hydrated, and keep making waves in your pursuit of a healthier, more active lifestyle.

Here's to your health and happiness, now and always! 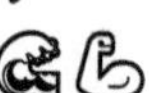

WORKOUT JOURNAL

DATE_______________________

MY WORKOUT

MY GOAL

MY NOTE

WORKOUT JOURNAL

DATE_______________________

MY WORKOUT

MY GOAL

MY NOTE

WORKOUT JOURNAL

DATE_______________________

MY WORKOUT

MY GOAL

MY NOTE

WORKOUT JOURNAL

DATE________________________

MY WORKOUT

MY GOAL

MY NOTE

WORKOUT JOURNAL

DATE_______________________

MY WORKOUT

MY GOAL

MY NOTE

WORKOUT JOURNAL

DATE________________

MY WORKOUT

MY GOAL

MY NOTE

WORKOUT JOURNAL

DATE ___________________

MY WORKOUT

MY GOAL

MY NOTE

WORKOUT JOURNAL

DATE_________________

MY WORKOUT

MY GOAL

MY NOTE

WORKOUT JOURNAL

DATE_______________________

MY WORKOUT

MY GOAL

MY NOTE

WORKOUT JOURNAL

DATE_______________________

MY WORKOUT

MY GOAL

MY NOTE